2019

This Diary/Planner Belongs To:

____

2019

January

S	M	T	W	T	F	S
30	31	1	2	3	4	5
6	7	8	9	10	11	12
13	14	15	16	17	18	19
20	21	22	23	24	25	26
27	28	29	30	31	1	2

February

S	M	T	W	T	F	S
27	28	29	30	31	1	2
3	4	5	6	7	8	9
10	11	12	13	14	15	16
17	18	19	20	21	22	23
24	25	26	27	28	1	2

March

S	M	T	W	T	F	S
24	25	26	27	28	1	2
3	4	5	6	7	8	9
10	11	12	13	14	15	16
17	18	19	20	21	22	23
24	25	26	27	28	29	30
31	1	2	3	4	5	6

April

S	M	T	W	T	F	S
31	1	2	3	4	5	6
7	8	9	10	11	12	13
14	15	16	17	18	19	20
21	22	23	24	25	26	27
28	29	30	1	2	3	4

May

S	M	T	W	T	F	S
28	29	30	1	2	3	4
5	6	7	8	9	10	11
12	13	14	15	16	17	18
19	20	21	22	23	24	25
26	27	28	29	30	31	1

June

S	M	T	W	T	F	S
26	27	28	29	30	31	1
2	3	4	5	6	7	8
9	10	11	12	13	14	15
16	17	18	19	20	21	22
23	24	25	26	27	28	29
30	1	2	3	4	5	6

July

S	M	T	W	T	F	S
30	1	2	3	4	5	6
7	8	9	10	11	12	13
14	15	16	17	18	19	20
21	22	23	24	25	26	27
28	29	30	31	1	2	3

August

S	M	T	W	T	F	S
28	29	30	31	1	2	3
4	5	6	7	8	9	10
11	12	13	14	15	16	17
18	19	20	21	22	23	24
25	26	27	28	29	30	31

September

S	M	T	W	T	F	S
1	2	3	4	5	6	7
8	9	10	11	12	13	14
15	16	17	18	19	20	21
22	23	24	25	26	27	28
29	30	1	2	3	4	5

October

S	M	T	W	T	F	S
29	30	1	2	3	4	5
6	7	8	9	10	11	12
13	14	15	16	17	18	19
20	21	22	23	24	25	26
27	28	29	30	31	1	2

November

S	M	T	W	T	F	S
27	28	29	30	31	1	2
3	4	5	6	7	8	9
10	11	12	13	14	15	16
17	18	19	20	21	22	23
24	25	26	27	28	29	30

December

S	M	T	W	T	F	S
1	2	3	4	5	6	7
8	9	10	11	12	13	14
15	16	17	18	19	20	21
22	23	24	25	26	27	28
29	30	31	1	2	3	4

2020

January

S	M	T	W	T	F	S
29	30	31	1	2	3	4
5	6	7	8	9	10	11
12	13	14	15	16	17	18
19	20	21	22	23	24	25
26	27	28	29	30	31	1

February

S	M	T	W	T	F	S
26	27	28	29	30	31	1
2	3	4	5	6	7	8
9	10	11	12	13	14	15
16	17	18	19	20	21	22
23	24	25	26	27	28	29

March

S	M	T	W	T	F	S
1	2	3	4	5	6	7
8	9	10	11	12	13	14
15	16	17	18	19	20	21
22	23	24	25	26	27	28
29	30	31	1	2	3	4

April

S	M	T	W	T	F	S
29	30	31	1	2	3	4
5	6	7	8	9	10	11
12	13	14	15	16	17	18
19	20	21	22	23	24	25
26	27	28	29	30	1	2

May

S	M	T	W	T	F	S
26	27	28	29	30	1	2
3	4	5	6	7	8	9
10	11	12	13	14	15	16
17	18	19	20	21	22	23
24	25	26	27	28	29	30
31	1	2	3	4	5	6

June

S	M	T	W	T	F	S
31	1	2	3	4	5	6
7	8	9	10	11	12	13
14	15	16	17	18	19	20
21	22	23	24	25	26	27
28	29	30	1	2	3	4

July

S	M	T	W	T	F	S
28	29	30	1	2	3	4
5	6	7	8	9	10	11
12	13	14	15	16	17	18
19	20	21	22	23	24	25
26	27	28	29	30	31	1

August

S	M	T	W	T	F	S
26	27	28	29	30	31	1
2	3	4	5	6	7	8
9	10	11	12	13	14	15
16	17	18	19	20	21	22
23	24	25	26	27	28	29
30	31	1	2	3	4	5

September

S	M	T	W	T	F	S
30	31	1	2	3	4	5
6	7	8	9	10	11	12
13	14	15	16	17	18	19
20	21	22	23	24	25	26
27	28	29	30	1	2	3

October

S	M	T	W	T	F	S
27	28	29	30	1	2	3
4	5	6	7	8	9	10
11	12	13	14	15	16	17
18	19	20	21	22	23	24
25	26	27	28	29	30	31

November

S	M	T	W	T	F	S
1	2	3	4	5	6	7
8	9	10	11	12	13	14
15	16	17	18	19	20	21
22	23	24	25	26	27	28
29	30	1	2	3	4	5

December

S	M	T	W	T	F	S
29	30	1	2	3	4	5
6	7	8	9	10	11	12
13	14	15	16	17	18	19
20	21	22	23	24	25	26
27	28	29	30	31	1	2

Important Dates/Events

2019 Goals

2019 Goals

2019 Goals

2019 Goals

January 2019

Monday	Tuesday	Wednesday
	1	2
7	8	9
14	15	16
21	22	23
28	29	30

Thursday	Friday	Saturday /Sunday
3	4	5/6
10	11	12/13
17	18	19/20
24	25	26/27
31		

February 2019

Monday	Tuesday	Wednesday
4	5	6
11	12	13
18	19	20
25	26	27

Thursday	Friday	Saturday /Sunday
	1	2/3
7	8	9/10
14	15	16/17
21	22	23/24
28		

March 2019

Monday	Tuesday	Wednesday
4	5	6
11	12	13
18	19	20
25	26	27

Thursday	Friday	Saturday /Sunday
	1	2/3
7	8	9/10
14	15	16/17
21	22	23/24
28	29	30/31

April 2019

Monday	Tuesday	Wednesday
1	2	3
8	9	10
15	16	17
22	23	24
29	30	

Thursday	Friday	Saturday /Sunday
4	5	6/7
11	12	13/14
18	19	20/21
25	26	27/28

May 2019

Monday	Tuesday	Wednesday
		1
6	7	8
13	14	15
20	21	22
27	28	29

Thursday	Friday	Saturday /Sunday
2	3	4/5
9	10	11/12
16	17	18/19
23	24	25/26
30	31	

June 2019

Monday	Tuesday	Wednesday
3	4	5
10	11	12
17	18	19
24	25	26

Thursday	Friday	Saturday /Sunday
		1/2
6	7	8/9
13	14	15/16
20	21	22/23
27	28	29/30

July 2019

Monday	Tuesday	Wednesday
1	2	3
8	9	10
15	16	17
22	23	24
29	30	31

Thursday	Friday	Saturday /Sunday
4	5	6/7
11	12	13/14
18	19	20/21
25	26	27/28

August 2019

Monday	Tuesday	Wednesday
5	6	7
12	13	14
19	20	21
26	27	28

Thursday	Friday	Saturday /Sunday
1	2	3/4
8	9	10/11
15	16	17/18
22	23	24/25
29	30	31/

September 2019

Monday	Tuesday	Wednesday
2	3	4
9	10	11
16	17	18
23 30	24	25

Thursday	Friday	Saturday /Sunday
		/1
5	6	7/8
12	13	14/15
19	20	21/22
26	27	28/29

October 2019

Monday	Tuesday	Wednesday
	1	2
7	8	9
14	15	16
21	22	23
28	29	30

Thursday	Friday	Saturday /Sunday
3	4	5/6
10	11	12/13
17	18	19/20
24	25	26/27
31		

November 2019

Monday	Tuesday	Wednesday
4	5	6
10	11	12
17	18	19
25	26	27

Thursday	Friday	Saturday /Sunday
	1	2/3
7	8	9/10
13	14	15/16
20	21	22/24
28	29	30/

December 2019

Monday	Tuesday	Wednesday
2	3	4
9	10	11
16	17	18
23	24	25

Thursday	Friday	Saturday /Sunday
		/1
5	6	7/8
12	13	14/15
19	20	21/22
26	27	28/29

December 2019/Janury 2020

Monday	Tuesday	Wednesday
30	31	1

Happy New Year!

December 2019|Janury 2020

Thursday	Friday	Saturday /Sunday
2	3	4/5

December

- 31. MONDAY

- 1. TUESDAY

- 2. WEDNESDAY

- 3. THURSDAY

- 4. FRIDAY

- 5. SATURDAY / 6. SUNDAY

Notes

January

○ 7. MONDAY

○ 8. TUESDAY

○ 9. WEDNESDAY

○ 10. THURSDAY

○ 11. FRIDAY

○ 12. SATURDAY / 13. SUNDAY

Notes

January

○ 14. MONDAY

○ 15. TUESDAY

○ 16. WEDNESDAY

○ 17. THURSDAY

○ 18. FRIDAY

○ 19. SATURDAY / 20. SUNDAY

Notes

January

○ 21. MONDAY

○ 22. TUESDAY

○ 23. WEDNESDAY

○ 24. THURSDAY

○ 25. FRIDAY

○ 26. SATURDAY / 27. SUNDAY

Notes

January

○ 28. MONDAY

○ 29. TUESDAY

○ 30. WEDNESDAY

○ 31. THURSDAY

○ 1. FRIDAY

○ 2. SATURDAY / 3. SUNDAY

Notes

February

- 4. MONDAY

- 5. TUESDAY

- 6. WEDNESDAY

- 7. THURSDAY

- 8. FRIDAY

- 9. SATURDAY / 10. SUNDAY

Notes

February

○ 11. MONDAY

○ 12. TUESDAY

○ 13. WEDNESDAY

○ 14. THURSDAY

○ 15. FRIDAY

○ 16. SATURDAY / 17. SUNDAY

Notes

February

○ 18. MONDAY

○ 19. TUESDAY

○ 20. WEDNESDAY

○ 21. THURSDAY

○ 22. FRIDAY

○ 23. SATURDAY / 24. SUNDAY

Notes

February

○ 25. MONDAY

○ 26. TUESDAY

○ 27. WEDNESDAY

○ 28. THURSDAY

○ 1. FRIDAY

○ 2. SATURDAY / 3. SUNDAY

Notes

March

- 4. MONDAY

- 5. TUESDAY

- 6. WEDNESDAY

- 7. THURSDAY

- 8. FRIDAY

- 9. SATURDAY / 10. SUNDAY

Notes

March

- 11. MONDAY
- 12. TUESDAY
- 13. WEDNESDAY
- 14. THURSDAY
- 15. FRIDAY
- 16. SATURDAY / 17. SUNDAY

Notes

March

○ 18. MONDAY

○ 19. TUESDAY

○ 20. WEDNESDAY

○ 21. THURSDAY

○ 22. FRIDAY

○ 23. SATURDAY / 24. SUNDAY

Notes

March

- 25. MONDAY
- 26. TUESDAY
- 27. WEDNESDAY
- 28. THURSDAY
- 29. FRIDAY
- 30. SATURDAY / 31. SUNDAY

Notes

April

- ○ 1. MONDAY
- ○ 2. TUESDAY
- ○ 3. WEDNESDAY
- ○ 4. THURSDAY
- ○ 5. FRIDAY
- ○ 6. SATURDAY / 7. SUNDAY

Notes

April

- 8. MONDAY

- 9. TUESDAY

- 10. WEDNESDAY

- 11. THURSDAY

- 12. FRIDAY

- 13. SATURDAY / 14. SUNDAY

Notes

April

- ○ 15. MONDAY
- ○ 16. TUESDAY
- ○ 17. WEDNESDAY
- ○ 18. THURSDAY
- ○ 19. FRIDAY
- ○ 20. SATURDAY / 21. SUNDAY

Notes

April

- [ ] 22. MONDAY

- [ ] 23. TUESDAY

- [ ] 24. WEDNESDAY

- [ ] 25. THURSDAY

- [ ] 26. FRIDAY

- [ ] 27. SATURDAY / 28. SUNDAY

Notes

April

- 29. MONDAY

- 30. TUESDAY

- 1. WEDNESDAY

- 2. THURSDAY

- 3. FRIDAY

- 4. SATURDAY / 5. SUNDAY

Notes

May

○ 6. MONDAY

○ 7. TUESDAY

○ 8. WEDNESDAY

○ 9. THURSDAY

○ 10. FRIDAY

○ 11. SATURDAY / 12. SUNDAY

Notes

May

- 13. MONDAY

- 14. TUESDAY

- 15. WEDNESDAY

- 16. THURSDAY

- 17. FRIDAY

- 18. SATURDAY / 19. SUNDAY

Notes

May

- 20. MONDAY
- 21. TUESDAY
- 22. WEDNESDAY
- 23. THURSDAY
- 24. FRIDAY
- 25. SATURDAY / 26. SUNDAY

Notes

May

○ 27. MONDAY

○ 28. TUESDAY

○ 29. WEDNESDAY

○ 30. THURSDAY

○ 31. FRIDAY

○ 1. SATURDAY / 2. SUNDAY

Notes

June

- 3. MONDAY

- 4. TUESDAY

- 5. WEDNESDAY

- 6. THURSDAY

- 7. FRIDAY

- 8. SATURDAY / 9. SUNDAY

Notes

June

○ 10. MONDAY

○ 11. TUESDAY

○ 12. WEDNESDAY

○ 13. THURSDAY

○ 14. FRIDAY

○ 15. SATURDAY / 16. SUNDAY

Notes

June

○ 17. MONDAY

○ 18. TUESDAY

○ 19. WEDNESDAY

○ 20. THURSDAY

○ 21. FRIDAY

○ 22. SATURDAY / 23. SUNDAY

Notes

June

○ 24. MONDAY

○ 25. TUESDAY

○ 26. WEDNESDAY

○ 27. THURSDAY

○ 28. FRIDAY

○ 29. SATURDAY / 30. SUNDAY

Notes

July

- 1. MONDAY
- 2. TUESDAY
- 3. WEDNESDAY
- 4. THURSDAY
- 5. FRIDAY
- 6. SATURDAY / 7. SUNDAY

Notes

July

- 8. MONDAY
- 9. TUESDAY
- 10. WEDNESDAY
- 11. THURSDAY
- 12. FRIDAY
- 13. SATURDAY / 14. SUNDAY

Notes

July

○ 15. MONDAY

○ 16. TUESDAY

○ 17. WEDNESDAY

○ 18. THURSDAY

○ 19. FRIDAY

○ 20. SATURDAY / 21. SUNDAY

Notes

July

- [ ] 22. MONDAY

- [ ] 23. TUESDAY

- [ ] 24. WEDNESDAY

- [ ] 25. THURSDAY

- [ ] 26. FRIDAY

- [ ] 27. SATURDAY / 28. SUNDAY

Notes

July

- 29. MONDAY

- 30. TUESDAY

- 31. WEDNESDAY

- 1. THURSDAY

- 2. FRIDAY

- 3. SATURDAY / 4. SUNDAY

Notes

August

- 5. MONDAY

- 6. TUESDAY

- 7. WEDNESDAY

- 8. THURSDAY

- 9. FRIDAY

- 10. SATURDAY / 11. SUNDAY

Notes

August

○ 12. MONDAY

○ 13. TUESDAY

○ 14. WEDNESDAY

○ 15. THURSDAY

○ 16. FRIDAY

○ 17. SATURDAY / 18. SUNDAY

Notes

August

○ 19. MONDAY

○ 20. TUESDAY

○ 21. WEDNESDAY

○ 22. THURSDAY

○ 23. FRIDAY

○ 24. SATURDAY / 25. SUNDAY

Notes

August

○ 26. MONDAY

○ 27. TUESDAY

○ 28. WEDNESDAY

○ 29. THURSDAY

○ 30. FRIDAY

○ 31. SATURDAY / 1. SUNDAY

Notes

September

- ○ 2. MONDAY
- ○ 3. TUESDAY
- ○ 4. WEDNESDAY
- ○ 5. THURSDAY
- ○ 6. FRIDAY
- ○ 7. SATURDAY / 8. SUNDAY

Notes

September

- ○ 9. MONDAY
- ○ 10. TUESDAY
- ○ 11. WEDNESDAY
- ○ 12. THURSDAY
- ○ 13. FRIDAY
- ○ 14. SATURDAY / 15. SUNDAY

Notes

September

○ 16. MONDAY

○ 17. TUESDAY

○ 18. WEDNESDAY

○ 19. THURSDAY

○ 20. FRIDAY

○ 21. SATURDAY / 22. SUNDAY

Notes

September

○ 23. MONDAY

○ 24. TUESDAY

○ 25. WEDNESDAY

○ 26. THURSDAY

○ 27. FRIDAY

○ 28. SATURDAY / 29. SUNDAY

Notes

September

- ○ 30. MONDAY
- ○ 1. TUESDAY
- ○ 2. WEDNESDAY
- ○ 3. THURSDAY
- ○ 4. FRIDAY
- ○ 5. SATURDAY / 6. SUNDAY

Notes

October

○ 7. MONDAY

○ 8. TUESDAY

○ 9. WEDNESDAY

○ 10. THURSDAY

○ 11. FRIDAY

○ 12. SATURDAY / 13. SUNDAY

Notes

October

- 14. MONDAY

- 15. TUESDAY

- 16. WEDNESDAY

- 17. THURSDAY

- 18. FRIDAY

- 19. SATURDAY / 20. SUNDAY

Notes

October

○ 21. MONDAY

○ 22. TUESDAY

○ 23. WEDNESDAY

○ 24. THURSDAY

○ 25. FRIDAY

○ 26. SATURDAY / 27. SUNDAY

Notes

October

- 28. MONDAY

- 29. TUESDAY

- 30. WEDNESDAY

- 31. THURSDAY

- 1. FRIDAY

- 2. SATURDAY / 3. SUNDAY

Notes

November

- 4. MONDAY
- 5. TUESDAY
- 6. WEDNESDAY
- 7. THURSDAY
- 8. FRIDAY
- 9. SATURDAY / 10. SUNDAY

Notes

November

○ 11. MONDAY

○ 12. TUESDAY

○ 13. WEDNESDAY

○ 14. THURSDAY

○ 15. FRIDAY

○ 16. SATURDAY / 17. SUNDAY

Notes

November

- 18. MONDAY
- 19. TUESDAY
- 20. WEDNESDAY
- 21. THURSDAY
- 22. FRIDAY
- 23. SATURDAY / 24. SUNDAY

Notes

November

- 25. MONDAY
- 26. TUESDAY
- 27. WEDNESDAY
- 28. THURSDAY
- 29. FRIDAY
- 30. SATURDAY / 1. SUNDAY

Notes

December

- ○ 2. MONDAY
- ○ 3. TUESDAY
- ○ 4. WEDNESDAY
- ○ 5. THURSDAY
- ○ 6. FRIDAY
- ○ 7. SATURDAY / 8. SUNDAY

Notes

December

- 9. MONDAY
- 10. TUESDAY
- 11. WEDNESDAY
- 12. THURSDAY
- 13. FRIDAY
- 14. SATURDAY / 15. SUNDAY

Notes

December

○ 16. MONDAY

○ 17. TUESDAY

○ 18. WEDNESDAY

○ 19. THURSDAY

○ 20. FRIDAY

○ 21. SATURDAY / 22. SUNDAY

Notes

December

- 23. MONDAY
- 24. TUESDAY
- 25. WEDNESDAY
- 26. THURSDAY
- 27. FRIDAY
- 28. SATURDAY / 29. SUNDAY

Notes

December

- ○ 30. MONDAY
- ○ 31. TUESDAY
- ○ 1. WEDNESDAY
- ○ 2. THURSDAY
- ○ 3. FRIDAY
- ○ 4. SATURDAY / 5. SUNDAY

Notes

2020 Key Dates

2020 Key Dates

Notes

Notes

Notes

Notes

Notes

Notes

www.ingramcontent.com/pod-product-compliance
Lightning Source LLC
Chambersburg PA
CBHW071549220526
45469CB00003B/953
9781730995545